COPING WITH
Disruptive Behavior
IN GROUP CARE

COPING
WITH
Disruptive
Behavior
IN
GROUP
CARE

EVA M. RUSSO AND ANN W. SHYNE

RESEARCH CENTER
CHILD WELFARE LEAGUE OF AMERICA, INC.
67 IRVING PLACE, NEW YORK, NEW YORK 10003

Library of Congress Cataloging in Publication Data

Russo, Eva Manoff.
    Coping with disruptive behavior in group care.

    Bibliography: p.
    1. Group homes for children—United States.
2. Problem children—United States. I. Shyne, Ann W.,
1914-   joint author. II. Child Welfare League of
America. III. Title.
HV881.R88   362.7'32   79-23739
ISBN 0-87868-137-X

CHILD WELFARE LEAGUE OF AMERICA
67 Irving Place, New York, New York 10003

Current printing (last digit)
10 9 8 7 6 5 4 3 2 1

Printed in the United States of America

CONTENTS

Acknowledgments   1

Introduction   3

Method   5

Characteristics of the Facilities   7

Characteristics of the Population Served   21

Disruptive Behavior Among Residents   33

Methods of Coping With Disruptive Behavior   39

Respondents' Views on Behavior Management
   at Their Facilities   45

Summary and Discussion of Survey Findings   59

Notes and References   69

Appendix   71

   Selected Excerpts from the Survey Questionnaire

THE IMPETUS FOR this survey came from the preliminary work and
concern of William Dearin, then Field Consultant, and Gloria T.
Chevers, Director of Standards Development, at the Child Welfare League. Their questions about difficulties encountered
by agencies in coping with problematic behavior and concern
about how and in what circumstances certain methods for controlling behavior are used formed the basis for the questionnaire that was eventually employed in the research.

Other individuals in various departments of the League
also participated in reviewing the initial questionnaire and
discussing the survey findings; Kirk Bradford, Zelma Felten,
Carol Frank, Emily Gardiner, Jeffrey Hantover, Shelby Hayden,
Joseph Moore and Clara Swan made noteworthy contributions to
the project. Ralph Cordes discussed the findings with the
staff and presented his questions and conclusions during a
panel discussion of the survey results at the Annual Meeting
of the American Orthopsychiatric Association in Washington,
DC, in April 1979.

CWLA agency personnel, representing 144 group care facilities, completed a lengthy questionnaire and many added comments and materials specific to their individual philosophy
and practice. Betty Jones and John Dorsey of Brookwood Child
Care in New York City pretested the questionnaire and suggested improvements. Alex Cohen, of the Pleasantville Cottage
School, Pleasantville, NY, was host to the survey staff on a
visit to the school. Andrew Diamond, of the Vista Del Mar
Child Care Service in Los Angeles, and Gerald Lefkowitz,
representing the Pleasantville Cottage School, contributed to
the panel presentation sponsored by the AOA.

The research was conducted by Eva Russo, with the invalu-
able assistance of Anne Moore and Alan Reich. Supervision
and consultation were provided by Deborah Shapiro, CWLA
Director of Research, from the project's inception through
January 1979, and thereafter by Mary Ann Jones, current Director of Research, who was moderator for the presentation
and discussion at the AOA conference. Responsibility for
presentation of survey findings at the conference was carried by Eva Russo. The final report is a collaborative
effort on the part of Eva Russo and Ann W. Shyne, who was
CWLA Director of Research from 1968 to 1976.

"ALMOST ALL senior practitioners and administrators with whom we had contact stated that today's children were 'more difficult,' 'more disturbed,' 'harder to reach,' etc., than in the 'good old days.'" So said Morris Fritz Mayer in discussing recent developments in group care.[1] The increased use of noninstitutional alternatives (principally foster family homes) for children who can function in a family setting has led to the closing of many of the institutions designed for the care of "normal" dependent and neglected children and to the conversion of others into residential treatment centers. In the last few years the characteristics of residents in child care institutions, treatment centers and group homes are believed to have been altered further as a consequence of the attempt to divert children and youths from the juvenile justice system. This effort, given further impetus by the passage of the 1974 Juvenile Justice and Delinquency Prevention Act, focuses particularly on status offenders--children and youths whose offenses would not be considered crimes if committed by adults.

Serving aggressive and violent children, whether labeled delinquents, status offenders or emotionally disturbed, requires more staff, makes special demands on staff, and necessitates "the availability of nonpunitive measures of coercion, of limitation of the child's movements."[2]

In attempting to develop and implement such measures, adults responsible for the care and treatment of "difficult" children struggle with varying and sometimes conflicting needs. The individual must be considered within the context of the group living situation and the group is, to a greater or lesser degree, influenced by its relationship to the surrounding community. In some instances, efforts to establish and maintain controls can result in measures that carry the potential of doing harm.

Concern among CWLA staff and some member agencies about the effects on group care facilities of the new demands placed upon them and the adaptations made to meet those demands prompted the survey reported here. In conjunction with an effort to update standards for agencies serving children in institutional settings,[3] the research was viewed as part of the League's continuing commitment to investigate emerging problems in services to children. In this instance the issues are specific to the incidence and management of disruptive behavior in group care. Questions were raised concerning the characteristics of the current populations in

3

child care institutions, residential treatment centers and group homes, and their impact on the nature and degree of problematic behavior at these facilities. In addition, information was sought about the location, size, program, staffing, etc., of the residences, as well as the incidence of disruptive behaviors and the methods employed in coping with them. It was hoped that the gathering of this information from a group of residential facilities would provide a comprehensive picture of the dilemmas and solutions involved in attempting to influence the behavior of troubled children and adolescents in group settings.

4

IN MAY 1978 a long questionnaire was sent to 168 League member agencies whose services were believed to include one or more of the following: group home service, institutional care, residential treatment. Each agency was asked to complete a separate qur stionnaire for each type of facility under its aegis. If an agency had more than one facility of a particular type (e.g., four or five group homes) it was asked to select one facility representative of that type. Responsibility for filling out the questionnaire was to be assigned to a senior staff person familiar with the daily administration of the facility as well as with agency policies and procedures.

Ten of the 168 agencies receiving the questionnaire indicated that they did not operate any residential facilities. These included eight public agencies that provide residential group care through purchase of service. Responses were received from 113 or 72% of the remaining 158 agencies queried. The replies related to 144 facilities--59 group homes, 16 child care institutions and 69 residential treatment centers, as classified by the respondents. Eighty-two agencies reported for a single facility, and 31 responded for two facilities, a group home and either a child care institution or a residential treatment center.

GENERAL DESCRIPTION

EACH OF THE NINE United States census regions and Canada was represented in the facilities from which completed question-naires were received. Nearly a fourth (34), however, were situated in the East North Central States (Illinois, Indiana, Michigan, Ohio and Wisconsin). The Middle Atlantic States (New Jersey, New York and Pennsylvania) ranked second in number of respondents, with 20 of the 144 facilities.

Nearly 81% (116) of all the facilities were under volun-tary auspices. Of these, three-fourths were nonsectarian and one-fourth sectarian. Nineteen percent (28) of the facili-ties were under public auspices. Table 1 shows the number and percent of group homes, child care institutions and resi-dential treatment centers in the public and voluntary sectors.

The length of time the facilities had provided their current type of care ranged from less than 1 year to more than 50 years, with 12.5 years the median.* Twelve facilities, most of which had been in existence for more than 50 years, had at some time changed their type of care, usually convert-ing a child care institution into a residential treatment center.

Nearly all of the facilities were described as located in urban and suburban (or small town) areas (94 urban, 42 sub-urban) and six were in rural areas. A large majority (101) described themselves as community-based, with the rest located on a campus; however, the latter were usually within three blocks of the nearest residential community. Practically all of the group homes (97%) were community-based, as were more than half (57%) of the residential treatment centers. Child care institutions were more likely to be located on a campus, with only 36% of these reported as community-based. Half the institutional and residential treatment facilities described their living arrangements as cottages, about a fourth de-scribed them as dormitories, and about a fourth as "apartment-like" units.

---

*Note: The median is the point that divides the sample in half when all the relevant numbers are ranked from lowest to highest. Fifty percent of the sample falls above the median and 50% falls below.

TABLE 1

Type of Facility by Auspices

| Type of Facility | Public | | Voluntary | | | |
| | | | Sectarian | | Nonsectarian | |
	%	No.	%	No.	%	No.
Group home	47	13	37	11	41	35
Child care institution	21	6	13	4	7	6
Residential treatment center	32	9	50	15	52	45
Total	100	28	100	30	100	86

Table 2 shows the number of current residents in each type of facility, and in the total sample. The median number of current residents for all types of facility was 18.4, but 18 (13%) had from 50 to 99 residents and nine (6%) had at least 100 residents. Child care institutions tended to have larger populations. The median number of current residents for child care institutions was 40, for treatment centers 34.5, and for group homes 6.9. More than two-thirds of the facilities (99) reported no substantial change over the last 5 years in the number of children and youths in residence. Twenty-five respondents (18%) reported an increase, and 18 (13%) a decrease.

Usual length of stay for residents in all facilities answering this question varied from under 6 months (11%) to 3 years or more (7%). The child care institutions reported the shortest length of stay, their median being 9 months. For both group homes and residential treatment centers the median length of stay was 15 months. The usual length of stay for all types of facility is reported in Table 3.

STAFF

Child care workers were the largest component of staff. The median number of child care workers employed by all facilities was nine. Ten respondents reported employing more than 50 child care workers. The median number of residents per child care worker for all facilities was 5.5 and the modal number of residents per child care worker, that is, the number occurring most frequently, was four. Table 4 indicates the number of residents per child care worker according to type of facility. Group homes had more child care workers per resident than either of the other two types of facility and, somewhat unexpectedly, residential treatment centers were found to have more residents per child care worker than either the group homes or the institutions.

Inquiries concerning the educational level of child care workers revealed a spread of formal schooling that ran the gamut from less than high school education to completed graduate degrees. As shown in Table 5, over one-third of the child care workers in 1977 were college graduates. An additional 54% were high school graduates, many with some college education short of graduation. Very few child care workers were at the extremes of having either less than a high school education or some graduate education. Table 5 also reveals that child care workers in the group homes and residential treatment centers in our sample tend to have higher levels of education than do the workers in the institutions.

9

TABLE 2

Number of Current Residents in the Facilities

Number of Current Residents	Child Care Institution (N = 16) %	Residential Treatment (N = 69) %	Group Home (N = 59) %	All Facilities (N = 144) %
Less than 10	--	4	72	32
10-19	25	17	28	22
20-49	37	48	--	27
50-99	19	22	--	13
100 and over	18	8	--	6
Median number of residents	40.0	34.5	6.9	18.4

TABLE 3

Usual Length of Stay in the Facilities

Length of Stay	Child Care Institution (N = 15) %	Residential Treatment (N = 69) %	Group Home (N = 58) %	All Facilities (N = 142) %
Under 6 months	20	13	7	11
6 months-11 months	53	23	33	30
1-2 years	14	42	30	35
2-3 years	13	13	22	17
3 years and over	--	9	7	7
Median length of stay (months)	9.0	15.0	15.0	15.6

TABLE 4

Number of Residents Served per Child Care Worker

No. of Residents per Child Care Worker	Child Care Institution (N = 14) %	Residential Treatment (N = 63) %	Group Home (N = 52) %	All Facilities (N = 129) %
1-3	21	26	34	28
4-6	50	38	44	41
7-9	7	20	20	18
10 and over	21	16	2	11
Median number of residents per child care worker	5.2	5.9	4.9	5.5

12

TABLE 5

Educational Attainment of Child Care Workers

| | Percentage of Child Care Workers | | | |
	Group Homes (N = 246)	Residential Treatment Centers (N = 1521)	Insti- tutions (N = 547)	Total (N = 2314)
Less than high school education	5%	2%	9%	4%
High school graduate	22	29	38	30
Some college education	19	24	25	24
College graduate	42	40	23	36
Some graduate education	9	4	3	4
Completed graduate degree	3	1	2	2

Over 80% of the facilities indicated that all child care workers received formal inservice training sponsored by the facility, most commonly through seminars and meetings. About one facility in 10 reported that at least half its child care workers had taken child care courses other than inservice training.

Of the 125 facilities that estimated the percentage of child care workers who left the facility in the course of any one year (see Table 6), 76 said less than 30% left, 25 reported a loss of between 30% and 50%, and the remaining 24 gave a figure of 50% or higher.

The second most numerous staff category reported was social workers. All but eight of the 139 facilities that responded to this question had at least one social worker on staff. (The eight facilities that had none used social workers from the rest of the agency or from the community.) The median number of social workers employed was two, and the median number of residents per social worker in facilities with any social workers was 12.

The proportions of facilities employing any staff in other categories were as follows:

Social work supervisor	74%	Nurse	30%
Child care supervisor	63%	Recreation worker	27%
Psychiatrist	55%	Physician	16%
Psychologist	38%	Dentist	3%
Teacher	38%	Education Director	3%

Sixty-two facilities or 44% reported that they had increased their staffs over the last 5 years, while only nine (6%) had reduced the number employed.

SERVICES AVAILABLE TO RESIDENTS

Table 7 lists 19 services in order of the frequency of their availability either at the facilities or in their communities. Schooling (including remedial or special education), recreation, individual casework, and medical and dental care were provided by almost all facilities (97% or more), usually to all residents. Sex education, group work (such as discussion or rap groups or resident committees), and family casework were also available in more than 90% of the facilities, but they were less likely than the first four listed to be provided to all residents.

14

TABLE 6

Child Care Worker Turnover

Annual Turnover Rate	Percentage of Facilities (N = 125) %
Under 20%	31
20%-29%	30
30%-49%	20
50% and over	19

TABLE 7

Services Available to Residents

(Percentage of Facilities*)

Schooling (including remedial and special education)	100%
Recreational/cultural activities	99
Individual casework	98
Medical care	97
Dental care	97
Sex/family life education	96
Group work	94
Religious services	93
Family casework	91
Aftercare	89
Individual psychotherapy	88
Formal diagnostic evaluation after admission	88
Physical education	84
Group psychotherapy	75
Vocational counseling	73
Vocational training courses	63
Formal diagnostic evaluation before admission	62
Vocational training on the job	61
Emergency shelter care	25

*The number responding for each service varied from 130 to 143.

16

At the other extreme were vocational training and formal diagnostic evaluation before admission, provided to residents in less than two-thirds of the facilities, and emergency shelter care, available in only one-fourth.

Of the 135 facilities responding to the question about schooling, 28% indicated that this was available at the facility, 35% in the community and 37% in both places. Schooling at treatment centers was about equally divided between facility only and both facility and community. For child care institutions, the response was usually "both," and for group homes it was "in the community." In addition to schooling, the services most likely to be provided in the community were vocational training, religious services, and medical and dental care.

In about three-fourths of the facilities some residents have an opportunity to work at the facility or in the community for pay. All the residents in two-thirds of the facilities and some of the residents in all but one of the others have an opportunity to participate in such community activities as visiting friends or joining Scout or Y groups. Such community participation on the part of all residents is, of course, more common in group homes than in congregate care settings. All of the facilities have provision for family visiting, usually both at the facility and elsewhere.

Asked whether any services had been discontinued in the last 5 years, 29 facilities or 20% replied in the affirmative. The services reported as discontinued were highly diversified, relating mostly to specialized programs such as summer camp. Two facilities had discontinued the provision of emergency shelter care. Financial constraints and lack of need were the principal reasons given for cutbacks in services.

The addition of new services was much more common, with 65% of the facilities reporting one or more additions. The services most often added--by 15 to 18 facilities--were psychological/ psychiatric service, remedial education/tutoring, recreational service and vocational service. Services added by six to 10 facilities were family casework, sex/family life education, on-ground schools, and aftercare. Only two facilities reported adding runaway shelters or arrangements for secure confinement.

Two-thirds of the facilities would like services not available at present. The services listed by more than five respondents as desirable additions were, in order of frequency, aftercare, vocational service, family service, day treatment, educational service/tutoring, intensive care unit/closed facility, and recreational program.

Some facilities responded to the questions regarding addition or deletion of services in terms of total agency programs. The program most frequently mentioned in this regard was group home service. Nine facilities reported that their agency had cut back on the number of group homes, six agencies had added this service, and 10 would like to see group homes provided by their agency.

REFERRAL SOURCES

For background for examining the specific characteristics of the children and youths coming into care, we were interested in the linkage between the facilities in the sample and other systems in relation to admission and discharge.

The major source of admission referral for almost all of the respondents was public child welfare agencies. Sixty percent (87) of the facilities received at least some referrals from this source. The median percentage of residents referred by public child welfare agencies was 57%, and in 17 facilities all the residents had been referred by public child welfare agencies. Police, courts and/or probation departments ranked second, but they were by no means a close second. Although 60% of the facilities received some referrals from these sources, the median percentage of current residents referred by the criminal/juvenile justice system was only 10%. Four facilities received all their referrals in this way. The percentage of facilities receiving any referrals from other sources was as follows:

Parents	44%	Diagnostic centers	25%
Voluntary agencies	34	Shelters	20
Psychiatric hospitals	32	Medical hospitals	12
Private physicians/ Psychiatrists	26	Self-referrals	9

Sixty-four percent of the facilities were usually able to admit residents within 1 month from the time of referral. In 12% of the facilities, admission was generally accomplished within 1 week. Twenty percent of the respondents reported a time lapse of from 1 to 3 months between referral and admission and the remaining 4% indicated a wait of up to 6 months or more.

Most of the respondents were either very well satisfied (28%) or somewhat satisfied (62%) with the amount and type of information usually received from the referral source at admission, with 10% not at all satisfied. The information found lacking by those who were not completely satisfied was most often family information, psychological or psychiatric data, medical data, and information on school performance and other current functioning. A few respondents expressed concern that lack of full information about prospective residents sometimes resulted in inappropriate admissions, leading, in some instances, to re-placement.

Asked how often it becomes necessary to discharge a resident permanently or temporarily because he or she is not adapting to the program, 94% of the sample answered "occasionally." Five facilities never find such discharge necessary, and three fre-quently do. The children or youths involved are most often dis-charged to public child welfare agencies, to parents, or to the criminal/juvenile justice system. Most of these discharges occur within a month of the decision to remove the resident.

Nearly two-thirds of the facilities reported that they oc-casionally find it necessary to admit or to keep children or youths who do not "belong" in the program, but only 3% are faced often with this situation. The reason cited is the lack of any other suitable resource for the residents in question.

As an addendum to the discussion on referral systems, it should be noted that the figures presented include some intra-agency transfers as well as referrals to and from "outside" systems (e.g., a resident might move from a treatment center or child care institution to a group home sponsored by the same public or voluntary agency). In these instances, respondents were usually more likely to be satisfied with information obtained at the time of admission.

19

WE INQUIRED about the age, race and ethnicity, income level, and intellectual, physical and emotional/behavioral characteristics of the residents in care during the years 1973 and 1977. Respondents were asked to estimate the proportion of their residents falling into listed categories during each of the designated years. Tables 8-13 are based on these approximate percentages. Most facilities were able to provide estimated statistics for 1977 in the various categories. Data for the earlier year were more difficult to obtain. The number of respondents for the 197⁻ data ranged from 119 to 129. Facilities in operation for less than 5 years (25) were instructed to substitute data from their first year for the 1973 percentages. Comparison of the data in terms of change over time revealed hardly any difference on most variables. Therefore, only the 1977 data are presented, except in instances where noticeable change occurred.

SEX AND AGE

About one-fourth of the facilities accommodate only girls, and a similar proportion accommodate only boys. In the 54% that serve both sexes, the composition is most often almost two-thirds boys.

Very few young children are residents in the child care facilities in this sample, as may be seen in Table 8. Three-quarters of the residents are adolescents, the largest group being in the 12-15 age bracket. In terms of type of facility it is interesting to note that the residents of the group homes tend to be older and the residents of the treatment centers tend to be younger when compared to the total sample of all residents.

RACE AND ETHNICITY

Nearly two-thirds of the residents in 1977 were white and over one-fourth were black (see Table 9). The remainder, less than 10% altogether, were composed of Hispanic and American Indian residents, with some children of other racial origins. The 16 institutions in the sample had a higher proportion of white residents and a lower proportion of black respondents than the other two types of facility. We do not know the extent to which the difference in the racial and ethnic distribution by type of facility is a reflection of the geographic distribution of the participating agencies.

21

TABLE 8

Age of Residents

| | Percentage of Residents | | | |
	Group Homes (N = 473)	Residential Treatment Centers (N = 3107)	Insti- tutions (N = 1171)	Total (N = 4751)
0-7 years	0%	4%	4%	4%
8-11 years	5	26	15	21
12-15 years	40	47	43	45
16 or over	55	23	38	30

TABLE 9

Race and Ethnicity of Residents

	Percentage of Residents			
	Group Homes (N = 473)	Residential Treatment Centers (N = 3209)	Institutions (N = 1171)	Total (N = 4853)
White	63%	61%	72%	64%
Black	26	30	18	27
Hispanic	4	6	7	6
American Indian	4	2	3	2
Other	3	1	0	1

The proportions of white and black populations showed some change over time, with the median percentage* of the white population in all facilities dropping from 81% in 1973 to 75% in 1977 and the median proportion of black residents increasing from 13% to 17%. A little more than one in five of the facilities reported no black residents in either year, while four facilities had all black youngsters in 1973, and three had all black residents in 1977. Ten percent of the facilities had all white youngsters in both years, while 3% had none.

INCOME LEVEL

Nearly half of all the residents in 1977 were considered to be from families living in poverty (see Table 10). An additional third of the residents were from low income families. Under 20% were from middle and upper income level families. The major difference by type of facility was between the poverty and low income residents, with the institutions reporting more poverty level children, the residential treatment centers reporting more low income level children, and the group homes at a midpoint between the other two types of facility.

The income level served in the designated years (1973 and 1977) was almost the same. Youngsters from low income groups remained predominant. There was, however, a small increase in the proportion of youths from middle and upper middle income families in residence from 1973 to 1977. The median percentage of middle income residents rose from 12% to 16%; and the upper middle income group, although still a small percentage of the total population, showed an increase in that 39% of the facilities reported the presence of some youngsters from upper middle class families in 1977, as compared with 31% in 1973. In Table 10 the income level distribution for 1977 residents is presented.

---

*Median percentage is the percentage that divides the sample in half. For example, one-half of all facilities in the sample reported that more than 75% of their residents in 1977 were white and one-half reported that less than 75% were white. This figure differs from those reported in Table 9 because the basis for median percentages is facilities (with all facilities weighted equally regardless of the number of residents), whereas the figures in Table 9 are based on residents.

TABLE 10

Income Level of Residents' Families

	Percentage of Residents			
	Group Homes (N = 466)	Residential Treatment Centers (N = 3068)	Insti- tutions (N = 1113)	Total (N = 4647)
Poverty level	52%	41%	64%	48%
Low income	28	39	21	34
Middle class	16	16	12	15
Upper middle class	4	4	3	3

INTELLECTUAL AND PHYSICAL FUNCTIONING

As may be seen in Table 11, 71% of the residents are reported to be average or above in intelligence. One-quarter are reportedly mildly retarded and 4%, moderately retarded. The residential treatment facilities reported more retarded children than did the other types of facility. A few of the respondents commented on the impact of emotional/behavioral disturbance on intellectual functioning--pointing out that some residents in the "mildly retarded" category might actually have average or above average capacity.

Even fewer of the residents were reported to have physical impairments, as may be seen in Table 12. Only 12% of the residents in 1977 were reported to have any physical disability and most of those were "mild." The institutions reported a somewhat greater number of physically disabled children than did the other two types of facility.

EMOTIONAL/BEHAVIORAL CLASSIFICATION

Table 13 reveals that 17% of the residents were classified as dependent/neglected at the time of admission. As expected, most of these children resided in the 16 child care institutions in the sample. A fifth of the residents were classified as "delinquent" and two-thirds were classified as having mild or severe emotional or behavioral disturbances. Not surprisingly, residential treatment centers reported a greater proportion of disturbed children than did the other two types of facilities. Nearly a third of the residents in the participating group homes and a quarter of the residents in the institutions were classified as delinquent.

The questionnaire called for the estimated percentage distribution of residents according to the four emotional/behavioral classifications at admission in 1973 and 1977. Although none of the differences between the two years is statistically significant, the responses lend some support to the impression of a decrease in the proportion of residents in care for reasons other than emotional/behavioral disturbance. The proportion of facilities reporting any dependent/neglected youngsters dropped from 55% in 1973 to 45% in 1977. On the other hand, although the percentage of facilities with any children reported as severely emotionally or behaviorally disturbed remained at about two-thirds, the median percentage of residents in this category increased from 10% to 17% from 1973 to 1977. Residents classified as delinquent were present in 57% of the facilities in 1973 and in 67% of the facilities in 1977. The median percentage of youngsters classified as delinquent rose from 6% in 1973 to 15% in 1977.

TABLE 11

Intellectual Functioning of Residents

	Percentage of Residents			
	Group Homes (N = 463)	Residential Treatment Centers (N = 3147)	Insti- tutions (N = 871)	Total (N = 4481)
Average and above	79%	67%	79%	71%
Mildly retarded	19	28	17	25
Moderately retarded	2	5	3	4
Severely retarded	0	0	1	0

TABLE 12

Physical Functioning of Residents

	Percentage of Residents			
	Group Homes (N = 473)	Residential Treatment Centers (N = 3147)	Insti- tutions (N = 1172)	Total (N = 4792)
No disability	90%	90%	83%	88%
Mild disability	9	9	16	11
Severe disability	1	1	1	1

TABLE 13

Emotional/Behavioral Classification of Residents

	Percentage of Residents			
	Group Homes (N = 473)	Residential Treatment Centers (N = 3178)	Insti- tutions (N = 1171)	Total (N = 4822)
Dependent/ neglected (a)	15%	8%	44%	17%
Mildly disturbed	32	38	26	34
Severely disturbed	22	38	6	29
Delinquent (b)	31	16	24	20

(a) Primary reason for placement not connected to child's behavior.

(b) Known to or referred by court because of antisocial behavior.

In examining the data concerning the emotional/behavioral characteristics of residents, one must keep in mind that (as with intellectual and physical functioning) the categories listed were broad and not precisely defined in the questionnaire. Further, since diagnostic classifications in these areas are subject to a good deal of variation, the results presented here should not be viewed as definitive indicators of the nature of the population served, but rather as broadly descriptive and somewhat impressionistic.

STATUS OFFENDERS

A separate series of questions concerned status offenders, that is, residents who, while they might be also classified as presenting varying degrees of emotional/behavioral disturbance, had committed offenses that would not be considered crimes had they been committed by adults. United States courts classify these youngsters as children, persons or juveniles "in need of supervision" for offenses such as incorrigibility, truancy, sexual promiscuity, use of alcohol, etc. Canadian classifications of juvenile offenders vary according to locality and do not necessarily approximate the status offender category. All respondents in this survey were given the foregoing definition of "status offender" as well as examples of offenses as an introduction to the questions concerning the presence of status offenders in their facilities.

Status offenders are admitted by 130, or 92%, of the 142 facilities that replied to these questions. The proportions accepting status offenders were almost the same in child care institutions, group homes and residential treatment centers. About three-fourths of the 130 facilities have accepted status offenders always, or at least since they adopted their present type of operation; the remaining one-fourth have accepted them only in the last few years. Only 14% of the 130 facilities indicated that they were required to accept status offenders by local, state or provincial regulation.

In view of the provision of the U.S. Juvenile Justice and Delinquency Prevention Act of 1974 for reimbursement to agencies through LEAA (Law Enforcement Assistance Administration) funds for service to status offenders, it is surprising that only 22 facilities indicated that their funding was "in any way dependent upon admission of this type of child."

The proportion of current residents considered by the responding agencies to fit our description of status offenders ranged from none (in five facilities) to all (in nine facilities), with a median proportion of 46% of the resident population. The median was almost identical in child care institutions, group homes and residential treatment centers. The proportion of youngsters currently in residence who had actually been adjudicated by the courts as status offenders was much smaller. The median percentage of adjudicated status offenders was 20, with little variation according to type of facility--group homes 23%, child care institutions 19% and treatment centers 18%.

In 93 facilities (74% of those facilities reporting the presence of status offenders), respondents said that their staff found the behavior of these youngsters to be no different from that of the rest of the resident population. Of the 36 that noted a difference, 18 described the status offenders as less responsive to restrictions and discipline, and 11 reported them as "acting out," being more assaultive or physically aggressive. On the other hand, five facilities reported their status offenders to be less problematic than other residents. They were described as having more control, being more mature and/or presenting fewer behavior problems in school.

It would appear that, for this sample, at this time, the youngster who would be classified as a status offender according to certain behavioral criteria is generally accepted by a sizable proportion of group care facilities. Many of these facilities have been admitting this type of youngster for years. The data do not indicate a sizable influx of status offenders as a result of court convictions or mandated placements as a consequence of recent legislation.

Approximately four-fifths of the facilities currently admitting status offenders do not view the behavior of this group to be more problematic than that of other residents. Data concerning the impact of the presence of status offenders on specific problematic behaviors is contained in the section of this report relating to disruptive behavior among residents.

CHANGES IN ADMISSION CRITERIA

In responding to a separate series of questions, 65 facilities (46%) reported that they had changed their admission policies within the last 5 years to admit certain types of youngster not previously accepted. The types of resident currently being admitted due to changes in policy in more than a single facility were: more disturbed (29 facilities); older youths (10); delinquents (9); status offenders (9); youngsters with lower IQs (9); younger children (6); and physically disabled youngsters (4). (Only changes in admission policies indicated by more than one facility are included here; some facilities reported more than one policy change.)

Forty-six of the 65 facilities indicated that these changes had been effected because of the increased need for service within a particular population. Fewer respondents reported that the changes in policy reflected changes in program or staffing (7), state policy (5), or the fact that funding was dependent on admitting such children (4).

Almost half (30) of the facilities that had expanded their admission criteria reported that administration and staff reacted favorably to these changes. One-fourth (17) required time to adjust to the change. In three instances the reaction was unfavorable, and in one it was necessary to hire different staff. In the remainder a mixed reaction or no reaction was reported.

Changes in policy to exclude certain groups of children and youths occurred less often than changes to extend admission criteria. Changes to restrict admission were reported by 28 facilities or 20%. The only categories mentioned by more than two respondents were younger children (5), aggressive youngsters (5), and older youths (3). The reasons commonly given for such exclusions were strain on the program (11) and change in program (8). The reaction of administration and staff was reported as usually positive (18), but in a few cases it was unfavorable or mixed (4), and in two instances staff changes were necessary.

The responses described here in respect to changes in admission criteria support, in a general sense, the population figures that show some increase in the proportion of residents who might be expected to engage in disruptive behavior. However, on an overall basis, substantial changes during this time period in regard to the type of population were not in evidence. Once again it seems as if the 1974 legislative mandate to divert certain juvenile offenders into the child welfare system has not had a dramatic effect on intake for the respondents in the survey at this time. One wonders if a review of the last 10 years might have provided greater evidence of a general increase in the number of older and more disturbed children and youths coming into care or if this effect might become more evident in the future.

THE SURVEY QUESTIONNAIRE listed 16 categories of disruptive behavior (see Appendix), with space provided for writing in any other type of behavior viewed as problematic by the staffs of the facilities. Respondents were asked to indicate whether "most," "some" or "none" of their present residents were involved in each behavior category. The majority of the respondents confined themselves to the list of behaviors on the questionnaire. Twenty-two facilities added other categories, the most common being severe depression/withdrawal (10 facilities).

Most of the behaviors listed were self-explanatory. Certain categories (e.g., loss of impulse control and inappropriate sexual behavior) were more subject to interpretation than others. In attempting to determine the incidence of problematic (or potentially problematic) behavior in the facilities, the perception of the respondents that a certain type of behavior was, in fact, occurring at their facility was considered important.

Of 16 behaviors listed on the questionnaire, all but fire setting and the use of drugs other than marijuana were reported by more than 75% of the facilities as involving at least some of their residents. Table 14 lists these behaviors in order of frequency of occurrence. As may be noted, verbal abuse, absence without leave, loss of impulse control and stealing occurred in 97% to 99% of the facilities responding to the questions on behavior.

Most of these disruptive behaviors were not pervasive among the residents. Only verbal abuse was reported for "most" residents by more than half the facilities (57%). Loss of impulse control was reported as prevalent in 22% of the facilities and use of marijuana in 16%. None of the other behaviors involved "most" residents in more than one facility in 10.

Facilities experiencing the behaviors were asked to indicate which of these had increased in the last 5 years. Table 15 shows the percentage of facilities that indicated an increase in the incidence of particular behaviors. Over half (56%) reported an increase in the use of marijuana, and almost half noted an increase in the use of other drugs (49%), physical abuse of others (45%) and verbal abuse of others (43%). The categories in which increases were least often reported by facilities faced with such behavior were stealing (28%), physical abuse of self (28%), hyperactivity (25%) and fire setting (20%).

TABLE 14

Incidence of Disruptive Behaviors Among Residents

Type of Behavior	Percent of Facilities Reporting*	
	Any residents involved in the behavior %	Most residents involved in the behavior %
Verbal abuse of others (143)	99	57
Absence without leave (143)	98	6
Loss of impulse control (143)	97	22
Stealing (143)	97	5
Refusal to cooperate in program (143)	94	7
Physical abuse of others (142)	94	10
Destruction of property (143)	93	10
Inappropriate sexual behavior (142)	89	8
Use of marijuana (139)	87	16
Refusal to go to school (140)	86	6
Hyperactivity (141)	86	5
Physical abuse of self (142)	81	--
Use of alcohol (142)	79	10
Disruption of community (143)	78	5
Use of other drugs (129)	67	3
Fire setting (142)	49	1

*Percentages are based upon the number of facilities responding to each question. Numbers are indicated in parentheses after each behavior category.

34

TABLE 15

Increase in the Prevalence of Disruptive
Behaviors in the Last 5 Years

Type of Behavior	Percent of Facilities Reporting an Increase*
Use of marijuana (121)	56
Use of other drugs (86)	49
Physical abuse of others (132)	45
Verbal abuse of others (140)	43
Destruction of property (133)	40
Use of alcohol (112)	39
Refusal to go to school (121)	38
Loss of impulse control (133)	35
Refusal to cooperate in program (132)	34
Absence without leave (138)	32
Inappropriate sexual behavior (126)	32
Disruption of community (110)	31
Stealing (137)	28
Physical abuse of self (113)	28
Hyperactivity (118)	25
Fire setting (69)	20

*Percentages are based upon the number of facilities answering
questions about an increase. Numbers are indicated in
parentheses after each category.

TABLE 16

Contribution of the Presence of Status Offenders to Increase in Disruptive Behaviors

Type of Behavior	Percent of Facilities Viewing Status Offenders as Contributing to Increase*
Refusal to go to school (46)	61
Refusal to cooperate in program (45)	60
Absence without leave (44)	57
Disruption of community (33)	52
Stealing (40)	50
Verbal abuse of others (57)	47
Physical abuse of others (53)	47
Destruction of property (49)	45
Inappropriate sexual behavior (39)	44
Use of alcohol (42)	38
Use of marijuana (65)	37
Use of other drugs (40)	32
Loss of impulse control (43)	30
Hyperactivity (28)	25
Physical abuse of self (30)	20
Fire setting (11)	18

*Percentages are based on the number of facilities reporting increased incidence of each behavior and answering the question on status offenders. Numbers are indicated in parentheses after each category.

Finally, respondents were asked if the presence of status offenders in the facility contributed to the reported increase in each behavior. Table 16 shows the percentage of facilities with reported increases that answered affirmatively. Increases in five behaviors were attributed at least in part to the presence of status offenders by half or more of those who answered: refusal to go to school; refusal to cooperate in the program; absence without leave; disruption of the community; and stealing. Status offenders were least likely to be regarded as contributing to increases in loss of impulse control, hyperactivity, physical abuse of self and fire setting.

In considering the total group of 130 facilities admitting status offenders, the proportion of respondents believing their status offenders to be influential in the increase of problematic behavior conformed to the small number (about one-fifth) who had stated earlier in the questionnaire that they believed these residents to be more disruptive than the rest of their population.

INQUIRY WAS MADE into the "usual" methods of coping with each of the behaviors and into procedures followed when the usual methods do not work and/or the situation becomes "acute." Nine possible methods were listed and described in the questionnaire, with opportunity for the respondents to specify other approaches (see Appendix). For the most part, the facilities were able to use the study's classifications. A common addition, "hospitalizing a resident," occurred because of incomplete definition of permanent or temporary discharge. When the questionnaires were edited, all hospitalizations (and the less frequently mentioned incarcerations) were coded under the "discharge" category. For the purposes of this study, a "discharge" was seen as any method of coping with a behavior or set of behaviors that involved removing a resident from the facility.

The responses in the "methods" section are not easy to summarize concisely, as facilities tended to check multiple methods for each behavior and as the methods vary with the circumstance and severity of the behavior. "Usual" and "acute" situations were dealt with (and no doubt defined by the respondents) differently. Here we try to note the most salient points.

One way of showing the relative application of different methods is by noting the frequency with which the various methods were employed in usual and acute situations. The highest possible frequency--2304--would occur if all 144 facilities mentioned the same method for all 16 behaviors (144 X 16). Since this did not happen, all the reported frequencies are less than that number.

USUAL SITUATIONS

Talk, including discussion of any sort with residents individually or in groups, was by far the most common approach in usual situations. This method was employed alone or in combination with other methods in response to every one of the behaviors listed except fire setting and destruction of property. The "talk" method was mentioned over 1600 times.

Second most common was *the withholding of privileges or the addition of chores or tasks*. This method was mentioned over 1000 times, or about two-thirds as often as talk. It was used by a substantial number of facilities for each behavior, but relatively less often in coping with physical abuse of self, inappropriate sexual behavior, hyperactivity and loss of impulse control.

Separation, or removal from the group, with or without the
company of a staff member, to a specified but *unlocked* place,
ranked third, noted 460 times. Separation was the most frequent
method other than talk in the case of physical abuse of others.
Two-thirds of the facilities employed separation for this behavior. It was used by about 40% of the facilities in dealing with
loss of impulse control, and by about 30% in coping with hyperactivity and verbal abuse.

Requiring the resident to make *reparation* for damages was
mentioned fourth (about 250 times). As might be expected, its
use was confined almost entirely to four behaviors: destruction
of property, stealing, disruption of the community, and fire
setting.

Physical restraint of the resident by one or more persons
in order to prevent harm to self, others or property ranked
fifth, with approximately 140 mentions. It was usually employed
in instances of physical harm to self or others and loss of impulse control.

Medication to alter behavior was rarely reported (50
mentions) as the usual method of handling problematic behavior.
All but three of the reported uses related to hyperactivity,
physical abuse of self or others and/or loss of impulse control.

Calling the *police* to subdue, arrest or locate a resident
(mentioned 42 times) was resorted to principally when a resident was absent without leave, but such action was reported by
only 23 of the 137 facilities that experienced this problem.
Three or four facilities usually call the police in instances
of community disruption, use of marijuana or other drugs, and
fire setting.

The only behaviors for which *discharge* (39 mentions) was
ordinarily used by more than three facilities were fire setting
(6), absence without leave (4), use of drugs other than marijuana (4), and use of alcohol (4).

Secure confinement in a locked room or unit is rarely the
usual response to any behavior. It was checked in all only 20
times as a usual procedure for: loss of impulse control (7);
physical abuse of others (4); fire setting (3); absence without
leave and physical abuse of self (2 each); and property destruction and hyperactivity (1 each).

In addition to the nine methods listed, only two others
were mentioned more than a handful of times. *Staffing,* or
assigning a staff member to stay with the child, was noted 30
times, mentioned by from one to four facilities for each of the
behaviors except verbal abuse, property destruction and steal-

ing. *A formal program of behavior modification* was mentioned 23 times--by from one to four facilities--for each of the behaviors except destruction of property and loss of impulse control.

ACUTE SITUATIONS

Except in the case of fire setting, the responses for dealing with acute situations present a very different pattern from that of methods in usual situations. Here *discharge* leads the list, with over 600 responses. At least 30 facilities use discharge in acute situations for every behavior except verbal abuse and hyperactivity.

Withholding privileges or assigning extra chores ranked second among methods for dealing with acute situations, reported a total of 390 times, and at least 10 times for every behavior except abuse of self and fire setting.

Separation, reported 284 times, ranked third, with the highest frequency for verbal abuse, physical abuse of others, and refusal to cooperate in the program. Resort to *police* almost as common as separation with 281 mentions, is used most often in acute instances of physical abuse of others, stealing, community disruption, absence without leave, and property destruction.

Talk --the most common approach in usual situations--was mentioned only 235 times in acute situations. In contrast to the pervasiveness of this method in usual situations of almost every behavior, in acute instances "talk" was employed primarily in cases of inappropriate sexual behavior; refusal to go to school; use of drugs, alcohol and marijuana; hyperactivity; and verbal abuse of others. A few facilities mentioned the use of representatives from Alcoholics Anonymous and drug rehabilitation programs for "talk" in situations of alcohol and other substance abuse.

Physical restraint, mentioned 205 times, is employed in acute situations for the same behaviors for which it is employed in usual situations, but somewhat more often. The same applies to *secure confinement* and use of *medication,* both reported much more often as emergency measures (about 135 times each) but in response to the same behaviors as in usual situations. *Staffing* was also used more often in crisis than in usual situations, but much less frequently than any of the methods already reviewed (49 mentions). *Reparations* for damages (61 mentions) and *application of a behavior modification program* (10 mentions), on the other hand, are less often used in acute situations than as a usual approach to disruptive behavior.

41

TABLE 17

Methods Most Often Used in Coping With Disruptive Behavior
in Usual and in Acute Situations

Type of Behavior	Usual Methods* No. of Facilities Responding	Usual Methods* Methods Most Often Used**			Methods in Acute Situations* No. of Facilities Responding	Methods in Acute Situations* Methods Most Often Used**		
Verbal abuse of others	139	98% Talk	42% Priv	29% Sep	109	63% Sep	40% Priv	12% Talk
Loss of impulse control	135	81% Talk	44% Sep	34% Priv	120	35% Phys	25% Dis	23% Med
Absence without leave	137	77% Talk	73% Priv	17% Pol	116	51% Dis	33% Pol	31% Priv
Stealing	137	89% Talk	69% Rep	64% Priv	104	38% Dis	38% Pol	28% Priv
Refusal to cooperate	134	91% Talk	54% Priv	23% Sep	106	42% Dis	35% Priv	25% Sep
Destruction of property	131	76% Rep	76% Talk	56% Priv	112	30% Dis	30% Pol	25% Phys
Physical abuse of others	130	70% Talk	67% Sep	42% Priv	120	56% Phys	40% Dis	37% Pol
Inappropriate sexual behavior	125	94% Talk	40% Priv	22% Sep	90	34% Dis	30% Talk	27% Priv
Use of marijuana	121	84% Talk	65% Priv	13% Sep	97	43% Dis	41% Priv	16% Talk
Refusal to go to school	119	92% Talk	66% Priv	14% Sep	92	39% Priv	36% Dis	30% Talk
Hyperactivity	116	67% Talk	34% Sep	21% Med	97	55% Med	18% Sep	14% 14% Talk/Dis
Physical abuse of self	113	93% Talk	30% Phys	19% Sep	103	50% Dis	47% Phys	20% Med
Use of alcohol	111	90% Talk	69% Priv	15% Sep	90	60% Dis	34% Priv	18% Talk
Disruption of community	107	79% Talk	77% Priv	30% Rep	93	41% Pol	37% Dis	26% Priv
Use of other drugs	88	88% Talk	70% Priv	18% Sep	75	65% Dis	27% Priv	19% Talk
Fire setting	63	95% Priv	75% Talk	27% Rep	63	65% Dis	21% Pol	14% Conf

*Conf = secure confinement Dis = discharge Med = medication Phys = physical restraint
Pol = police Priv = privileges Rep = reparation Sep = separation Talk = talk

** Percentages are based on the number of facilities responding. Percentages for a given
behavior frequently add to more than 100% because facilities reported more than one
method.

This discussion has focused on methods, with specific behaviors secondary. In Table 17 the focus is on behavior. The table shows the three methods most often reported as usual methods, and as methods used in extreme situations for 16 behaviors, with the percentage of facilities reporting each method used. For example, from the first line of Table 17 it may be seen that 98% of the facilities used *talk*, 42% *withholding of privileges* and 29% *separation*, alone or in combination with other methods, in dealing with nonacute verbal abuse. The same three methods were those most commonly used with verbal abuse in acute situations, but their order was different, with separation resorted to most often.

IN ADDITION TO the behavior and methods check lists, respondents were asked a series of open-ended questions regarding their overall judgment of the difficulty their staff was experiencing in coping with problematic behavior and methods found to be most and least successful. As to how problematic the facility found behavior management, the most frequent response was "moderate problem," given by 59%. The next largest group (29%) considered it a mild problem, and the remaining 12% judged it a severe problem. The responses from the group homes had the same distribution as those from child care institutions and treatment centers.

The behaviors found most difficult by staff were: aggressive/acting-out behavior, mentioned by 55%; assaultive behavior--46%; absence without leave/runaways--39%; drug use (including marijuana)--14%; depression/suicide attempts--12%; and inappropriate sex--11%.

Forty-two percent of the respondents stated that they were very well satisfied with the methods used in their facilities for coping with disruptive behavior. Most of the others (55%) were somewhat satisfied. There was no difference in the degree of satisfaction in the three types of facility. Ways of coping with disruptive behavior found most successful by the 135 respondents answering this question in their own words were:

	% (N = 135)*	No.
Restriction of privileges	41	(55)
Developing consistent relationships	35	(48)
Counseling	34	(46)
Separation from the group	24	(33)
Behavior modification/ rewards	15	(21)
Peer pressure	13	(17)

*Some facilities gave multiple responses to this question.

Interestingly, restriction of privileges also led the list of methods mentioned as least successful by the 121 respondents who answered the question.

Methods most frequently reported as least successful were:

	% (N = 135)*	No.
Restriction of privileges	24	(29)
Physical restraint	18	(22)
Inconsistency	16	(19)
Excessive talk/lecturing	16	(19)
Staff anger	15	(18)

The importance of planful intervention as well as relationships with staff (particularly child care workers) and with peers was emphasized in some of the narrative comments.

> We subscribe to the theory that behavior control begins with milieu, relationship and program activities, and the specifics (i.e., the methods listed on the questionnaire) and the control thereof are a view of behavior management in a narrow but very important sense.

> We have put a much greater emphasis on the nurturing role of the cottage staff. We have had to teach this to our mostly young (under 30) cottage staff, but it has appeared to pay off in a dramatic decrease in the amount of physical acting out and property damage since we have been doing it consistently.

> The staff is very flexible, secure and skilled at tolerating and handling the behavior of these very difficult children. Group intervention is very effective in changing behavior and is skillfully utilized by the staff.

> We believe that we have fewer behavior problems when we are planful, anticipate, and have good activity programming. There is also less acting out in cottages where the child care workers have all been with us over a year.

The use of medication in coping with problematic behavior was explored to a limited degree in the questionnaire. Excluded from the questionnaire were the nature of the medications used and their role within the total treatment plan.

Although medication was checked infrequently as the usual method of dealing with any type of behavior, 98 (69%) of the facilities had made some use of medication over the last 5 years to control or alter behavior (excluding its use with neurologically based seizure disorders). As mentioned in the previous section, medication was most frequently employed in controlling hyperactivity, both in usual and acute situations. It was often used but somewhat less frequently in instances of loss of impulse control and physical abuse of self. Tables 18 and 19 show the distribution of reported use of medication in usual and acute instances of different behaviors.

Use of medication was reported most frequently by residential treatment centers (78%) and least often by group homes (59%), with child care institutions in between (69%). Among the institutional settings (child care or treatment), those with 10 or more child care workers and those with two or more social workers more often reported use of medication. Medication was used less by the facilities under public auspices (46%) than by voluntary nonsectarian facilities (70%) or sectarian facilities (86%).

As might be expected, the higher the proportion of disturbed children, the more likely the facility was to report use of medication. The relation of the presence of many seriously disturbed children to use of medication is further evidenced by three other findings: medication was used by more facilities where the usual length of stay exceeded a year (77%) than where the usual stay was under a year (58%); it was used by more facilities with psychologists on the staff (79% versus 56%); and by more facilities with psychiatrists on staff (77% versus 50%). Medication was also employed by more of the facilities that had been accepting status offenders for at least 5 years than by other facilities (73% versus 45%). Reports of use of medication were more common from facilities that provide a formal preadmission and/or postevaluation of all residents. Many of these differences no doubt reiterate the greater use of medication in residential treatment centers compared with group homes and institutions.

TABLE 18

Facilities Reporting the Use of Medication
as a Method of Coping With Problematic Behavior
in Usual Situations

Type of Behavior	Number of Facilities*	Percentage of Facilities	
		Facilities Using Medication (N = 98)	All Facilities (N = 144)
Hyperactivity	29	30%	20%
Physical abuse of self	11	11	8
Loss of impulse control	10	10	7
Physical abuse of others	1	1	1
Refusal to go to school	1	1	1

*These totals include the use of medication as either the sole method or in combination with other methods.

TABLE 19

Facilities Reporting the Use of Medication
as a Method of Coping With Problematic Behavior
in Acute Situations

Type of Behavior	Number of Facilities*	Percentage of Facilities	
		Facilities Using Medication (N = 98)	All Facilities (N = 144)
Hyperactivity	53	54%	37%
Loss of impulse control	28	29	19
Physical abuse of self	22	22	15
Physical abuse of others	10	10	7
Fire setting	4	4	3
Inappropriate sexual behavior	4	4	3
Refusal to cooperate in program	4	4	3
Refusal to go to school	3	3	2
Use of alcohol	3	3	2
Use of drugs other than marijuana	2	2	1
Use of marijuana	1	1	1
Destruction of property	1	1	1
Absence without leave	1	1	1
Disruption of community	1	1	1

*These totals include the use of medication as either the sole
method or in combination with other methods.

Use of medication was also more prevalent among facilities that reported an increase in recent years in any of the following behaviors: physical abuse; destruction of property; disruption of the community; refusal to cooperate in program; absence without leave; use of marijuana or other drugs; use of alcohol and loss of impulse control. Facilities that considered aggressive/assaultive behavior more difficult than any other were more likely to employ medication, as were those where staff was not very well satisfied with its methods of handling problematic behavior.

Four-fifths of the facilities reporting the use of medication indicated that it had been used "rarely" in the last year. Almost another fifth used it "fairly often: and two agencies, "very often." The median percent of the resident population requiring medication in the last year was estimated as 18%.

Facilities that used medication and those that did not cited both advantages and disadvantages to its use. Of 112 respondents who commented on the advantages of using medication, 90 (80%) remarked on its value in controlling behavior or alleviating symptoms, and 36 (32%) noted that it made the child more alert and accessible. (These figures include 26 respondents who mentioned both these values.) Nine saw no advantages. The disadvantages most frequently cited were:

	% (N = 116)*	No.
Masks symptoms	38	(43)
Crutch for child	32	(36)
Produces side effects	30	(34)
Crutch for staff	22	(25)
Habit forming	17	(19)
Requires more trained staff	10	(11)

*Some facilities gave multiple responses to this question.

In addition to these disadvantages, other reasons for not using medication given by several of the 37 respondents not employing medication and answering the question were the lack of need for it in the population served (14) and its being contrary to the philosophy of the facility (17).

Of those facilities using medication in the last 5 years, most (57%) reported no change in the frequency of its use. Eighteen percent had increased its use because the facility had a more disturbed population. On the other hand, 25% had decreased the use of medication, usually because the staff had become more skilled, the population had become less disturbed, or the facility simply disliked this method.

It is usually child care staff alone or with other staff who request medication for the resident. The medication is always prescribed by a psychiatrist or other physician employed by the facility or familiar with the resident, most often by a psychiatrist. Monitoring the resident's reaction to medication is customarily the responsibility of the child care staff, although occasionally this responsibility rests with medical, nursing or psychiatric staff. The child care worker keeps a log in most instances, frequently meets with the psychiatrist and the team, and occasionally reports in writing to the psychiatrist. Authorization for continuance or discontinuance of medication ordinarily rests on periodic team review. In 22 facilities the review and final decision are left solely up to the psychiatrist.

In a third of the facilities using medication the governing board or advisory committee had discussed this practice, and in one instance general opposition was expressed. Twelve facilities had had complaints (usually from parents of residents) about the use of medication. These were handled by discussion with the complainant, and in one instance a complaint prompted a review of the procedures.

USE OF SECURE CONFINEMENT

About one-fifth (22%) of the 144 facilities (32) participating in this survey reported using secure confinement within the last 5 years. In usual situations (see Table 20) it was employed most frequently in coping with loss of impulse control. In more difficult situations the use of secure confinement covered a broader range of behavior categories (see Table 21). Behaviors most often mentioned as requiring confinement in acute situations were: physical abuse of others; loss of impulse control; destruction of property; absence without leave; and disruption of the community.

Only one of the 32 facilities using confinement said that it had been used very often in the last year; 12 said "fairly often," 17 "rarely," and two "not at all," as its use had been discontinued. Of the 26 agencies reporting the number of residents re-

TABLE 20

Facilities Reporting the Use of Confinement
as a Usual Method of Coping With Problematic Behavior

Type of Behavior	Number of Facilities*	Percentage of Facilities	
		Facilities Using Confinement (N = 32)	All Facilities (N = 144)
Loss of impulse control	7	22%	5%
Physical abuse of others	4	12	3
Fire setting	3	9	2
Physical harm to self	2	6	1
Absence without leave	2	6	1
Destruction of property	1	3	1
Hyperactivity	1	3	1

*Totals reflect use of confinement as the sole method or in
combination with other methods.

quiring secure confinement in the last year, the range was from none to more than 75% of the resident population.

In most instances, the place of confinement was described as a bare, locked room with adequate ventilation and access to toilet facilities. The procedure for monitoring a resident in confinement is usually to have a staff member check every 15 minutes and keep a written log. In a few facilities a staff member remains outside the door all the time, but in a few others the youngster is checked only at half-hour or longer intervals. The minimum period of confinement was most often described as "a few minutes" but a few facilities reported a minimum period of from 1 to 3 hours. Twelve facilities cited their maximum period of confinement as being under 6 hours, while another 12 said "24 hours or more." A detailed description of how confinement is used in one facility is given at the end of this section.

As in the case of medication, child care workers alone or with other staff are the persons likely to request that a resident be confined in a secure setting. Authorization for confinement most often rests with the executive director/administrator (12 facilities), but it may lie with the child care supervisor (6), psychiatric staff (5), child care staff (4), social work staff (2) or the team (2). In 21 facilities written authorization is required.

Comments on the advantages and the disadvantages of the use of secure confinement were received from 85 facilities, many of which do not employ this method of handling disruptive behavior. Forty-two respondents stated that confinement helps the child to regain control/calm down, and 39 felt that it prevents harm to the child or others. Some cited both of these advantages. Five noted that it avoids discharge. No advantages were perceived by 14 of the 85 who commented.

The principal disadvantages to secure confinement cited alone or in combination were: it may be abused by staff (41); it is psychologically harmful to the child (30); and it does not help to establish internal controls (27). Five of those responding to this question saw no disadvantages. The reasons for not using confinement mentioned most often by 95 respondents not employing this method were: confinement is against the philosophy of the facility (26); other methods are more effective (22); it is prohibited by state/local law (15); the population served does not require it (13); and the facility does not have a secure room/unit (13).

Of the 31 facilities responding to a question about change in the use of confinement over the last 5 years, five reported

TABLE 21

Facilities Reporting the Use of Confinement
in Acute Situations

Type of Behavior	Number of Facilities*	Percentage of Facilities	
		Facilities Using Confinement (N = 32)	All Facilities (N = 144)
Physical abuse of others	23	72%	16%
Loss of impulse control	21	66	15
Destruction of property	16	50	11
Absence without leave	15	47	10
Disruption of community	10	31	6
Fire setting	9	28	6
Physical abuse of self	7	22	5
Refusal to go to school	6	19	4
Refusal to cooperate in program	6	19	4
Hyperactivity	5	16	3
Verbal abuse of others	5	16	3
Inappropriate sexual behavior	4	12	3
Stealing	4	12	3
Use of drugs other than marijuana	3	9	2
Use of alcohol	3	9	2
Use of marijuana	2	6	1

*Totals reflect the use of confinement as the sole method or in
combination with other methods.

54

an increase, usually because of a more disturbed population. Eighteen facilities reported a decrease, in two instances because of a less disturbed population, and in 16 cases because other methods were found to be more effective.

Secure confinement was found to be employed much less often in group homes, of which only four (7%) had used it in the last 5 years, than in residential treatment centers (32%) or child care institutions (38%). Factors associated with the use of secure confinement in the congregate care facilities were examined. Group homes were dropped from the analysis, since the number using secure confinement was so small. Only a few differences large enough to be statistically significant were found between the 28 congregate care facilities that used secure confinement and the 56 that did not. Significantly greater use of secure confinement was found in congregate care facilities with more than two social workers on staff; with psychologists on staff; and with psychiatrists on staff. In general it appears that secure confinement is used more by facilities with a larger and more diversified treatment staff. There was also considerable overlap between the facilities using secure confinement and those using medication to control behavior. Twenty-eight (87%) of the 32 facilities that used secure confinement during the last 5 years also used medication, including three of the four group homes employing secure confinement.

Most of the 32 facilities using secure confinement had had discussions of this usage by their governing board or advisory committee. In all cases it was approved, although one facility reported that confinement was to be restricted to extreme cases.

About half the facilities employing this method of control had had complaints about the use of secure confinement, some from their own staff. Most of these were handled through discussion with the complainant. Three entailed formal grievance procedures, and one involved a state-supervised appeal.

A more detailed account of the use of secure confinement was provided by some of the participating facilities. Although not necessarily typical, the following is an example of secure confinement based on a description from one agency. It is presented to give the reader a closer look at factors involved in employment of this method.

This facility is one of the small percentage in the responding sample that believes the use of secure confinement to be beneficial. It is a residential treatment center, in operation for over a quarter of a century. Its "isolation unit" was instituted 5 years ago. The stated purpose for constructing this unit was to end the necessity for emergency hospitalizations. In addition to the fact that it was often difficult to have residents admitted to the hospital on this basis, it was felt that such a procedure was degrading to the individual and frequently produced a "revolving door syndrome" whereby a child came back to the facility more disturbed and heavily medicated. Since establishment of the isolation unit this facility has not had to admit anyone to a psychiatric hospital on an emergency basis.

Secure confinement is carried out in a self-contained locked unit on top of the infirmary building. In addition to toilet facilities, it consists of two rooms (windowed and bare except for a mattress) that can be locked, separated by an observation room that contains provision for staff to stay overnight and communicate with other staff by telephone. Originally the secure rooms were separated from the observation rooms by one-way mirrors. These were eventually replaced with plexiglass enabling residents to view staff. The windows to the outside are barred to prevent escape.

Initially there was concern about both abuse and acceptance by staff. In terms of acceptance, opponents and proponents of the unit came from all job categories. Communication as to the purpose of the unit and experience with its use resulted in gradual acceptance on the part of staff. To prevent abuse, certain safeguards were developed.

Staff are expected to adhere scrupulously to state guidelines in terms of reporting and writing up such items as the reason for and length of time in each use of the room. Regardless of who requests the use of the room, a unit administrator is responsible for the final decision in each case. Further, a member of the child care staff must be present at all times--either in the secure room itself or in the observation room, depending on the needs of the resident.

No maximum amount of time for stay is set--some residents stay more than 24 hours, often while awaiting planful discharge. The average length of stay is 4-5 hours. The unit was originally used exclusively for youngsters who were potentially dangerous to themselves or others, and gradually this use has expanded to include other youngsters who may become panicky or uncontrolled in their behavior. The use of the unit is seen usually, but not always, as a last resort. The procedure by which control and organization are established in this unit is to have the resident change into pajamas, make up the bed, and remove potentially harmful objects such as jewelry. As the resident gains self-control, reinforcement is provided in terms of returning his or her possessions.

Although employment of this unit is not seen as accomplishing the long-term integration of internal controls, it is regarded by this facility as useful in providing a safe environment, reducing the resident's sense of omnipotence, and decreasing crippling anxiety.

CHARACTERISTICS OF THE STUDY SAMPLE

RESPONSES FROM 144 group care settings affiliated with the Child Welfare League of America--59 group homes, 16 child care institutions and 69 residential treatment centers--furnished data on the facilities, their residents, the incidence of disruptive behavior, and the methods of dealing with it. A session at the Annual Meeting of the American Orthopsychiatric Association in April 1979 provided an opportunity to review the survey findings with knowledgeable child care people. Their responses contributed substantially to formulation of the views and recommendations in the closing section of this report.

Before consideration of the survey results, the limitations of the sample should be cited. The exclusive use of Child Welfare League member agencies restricted the respondent population to agencies that, while diverse, are expected to adhere to specified standards for group care of children. These agencies also undergo periodic scrutiny by the League's field consultants through reaccreditation studies. A sample of this type cannot be considered representative of group care facilities in general.

Another limitation is that the respondents were, for the most part, administrators or other senior personnel. The questionnaire yielded data on both the overall philosophy of the facilities and the practices outlined by administration and presumably adhered to by staff. The way in which line staff perceived the problems and carried out the methods described is often hinted at, but not known firsthand. It has been suggested that a similar survey of child care workers and other line staff (such as teachers) might prove fruitful,(4) both in adding another perspective to the perception of problem areas and in underlining differences (to the degree that they exist) between policy and practice.

The 144 facilities are widely scattered geographically. Most are under voluntary auspices and have been in operation for many years. On the average, group homes had seven residents, child care institutions 40, and treatment centers 34. Child care institutions reported the shortest length of stay--9 months on the average, compared with 15 months in the other two types of setting.

Child care workers represent the largest group of staff employed by the facilities. The median number of residents served per child care worker is 5.5. High school and college graduates predominate among the child care workers at the facilities. Almost all of the facilities provide inservice training for their child care workers, mostly in the form of seminars and meetings. Thirty-nine percent of the respondents reported that at least one-third of their child care staff leave the facility during the course of a year. Social workers are present in almost all of the facilities. The median number of residents served per social worker is 12.

Services most often provided by the facilities are schooling, recreation, individual casework, medical and dental care. Services least likely to be available to residents are vocational training and emergency shelter care.

Over half of the residents in most of the facilities had been referred by public child welfare agencies. The second most common source of referral was police, court or probation departments, although this source comprised only about 10% of all referrals for most facilities.

Almost all (94%) of the facilities occasionally have to discharge a resident who is not adapting to the program. The primary resources for discharge are public child welfare agencies, parents, and police, court or probation departments. Facilities sometimes keep children who are not adapting to the program, usually because no other suitable resource is available.

Children 12 to 15 years old predominate among the residents, with those 16 years and older the next largest group. About a fifth of the facilities have no black children; the median proportion of black residents across all facilities is 17%. The children come chiefly from poverty-level and working-class families. Most are of at least average intelligence and free from physical disabilities. In only a few facilities, however, do children free from emotional or behavioral disorders constitute a majority of the residents. Children with mild or moderate emotional disorders and delinquents represent substantial proportions of the residents in most of the facilities. In the typical agency 46% of the children could be considered status offenders according to behavioral definitions, but only 20% are actually adjudicated as status offenders by the courts. In most facilities the behavior of status offenders is seen as no different from that of other residents. It would appear, then, that while these facilities are indeed serving troubled children, the diversion of status offenders from the juvenile justice system into child welfare facilities has not yet had significant impact on the behavior management problems experienced at the facilities in this sample.

A wide range of disruptive behaviors was reported as exhibited by at least some of the residents in most facilities. Verbal abuse, loss of impulse control, absence without leave, and stealing are the most pervasive of these behaviors. Problematic behaviors most often reported as having increased in the last 5 years are use of marijuana, use of other drugs, physical abuse of others and verbal abuse of others.

"Talk," restriction of privileges, and separation of the child from the group to an unlocked place far outrank other methods of dealing with disruptive behavior in usual situations, but discharge is by far the most common response in acute situations.

Over 70% of the facilities consider the management of problematic behavior at their facility to be at least a moderate problem. Most are somewhat but not fully satisfied with their ways of coping with disruptive behavior. Differences of opinion about what works best are well illustrated by the fact that restriction of privileges is the method most frequently reported as both *most* and *least* successful.

In a survey of this type, the bulk of the findings represents a statistical summary of descriptive data about both residents and staff, together with overall impressions concerning severity of problems and satisfactory solutions. Information on the quality of individual and group behavioral interactions is more difficult to obtain, but should not be overlooked in considering the factors contributing to disruptive behavior. For example, if a particular behavior is experienced by an individual or group as an irritant or seriously disruptive, then the behavior itself (and often the individual engaging in it) becomes classified as problematic. As mentioned earlier in the report, most behaviors are difficult to define precisely on a broad scale and are also subject to the perceptions, tolerance and value systems of administrators, staff and residents. Within this framework there was a common base of agreement among respondents concerning the potential hazards posed by some behaviors as opposed to others (verbal abuse is generally tolerated within certain limits; fire setting is most often viewed with gravity). What we cannot determine from this type of datum is the potential for escalating or provoking crises of the seemingly benign behaviors.

Consider, for instance, "verbal abuse of others," the most prevalent of the behaviors, and one of those reported as having increased over the last 5 years. This behavior is handled primarily in both "usual" and "acute" instances by talk, separation and restriction of privileges. There are, of course, variations here--in fact five of the facilities employ secure confinement for acute verbal abuse. It would appear, though, from survey results that, for the most part, verbal abuse is viewed as relatively innocuous behavior, not likely to present physical danger to oneself or others. In thinking about the realities of daily interaction between residents and staff, however, one might examine the part played by verbal abuse or other irritating behavior in relation to other, less controlled, physically active outbursts. It is conceivable that at a certain point, severe or sustained verbal abuse or other types of provocation can escalate into more violent reactions on the part of residents and/ or staff.

Similarly, examination of the numerous possibilities inherent in the definition of methods of coping with problematic behavior both points to the need for more specific information and offers some possible explanation for certain discrepancies in the findings. A pertinent example here is "restriction of privileges," a method reported frequently for a variety of behaviors, heading the lists of both the "most" and "least" successful ways of coping with problematic behavior. A few of the questions raised in reviewing the data regarding "restriction of privileges" were: What constitutes such restriction within a particular facility for a particular behavior engaged in by a particular resident? (Possibilities could range from missing a TV program to being denied a weekend family visit.) Is this method applied in a consistent manner? Does the degree of restriction or assignment of extra tasks conform to the nature and severity of the behavior? Is the intent and application of the prohibition punitive? Given speculation on these questions and others, it becomes easier to understand why this method, while frequently used, appeared to be so controversial.

In considering methods of control that might have harmful effects, none is really exempt. For instance, just as verbal abuse by residents has the potential for leading to severe disruption, so does the "talk" method of handling behavior that is employed so frequently and variously by the responding facilities. Obviously, what we do not know here is who is doing the talking, what is being said and in what tone of voice the communication is delivered. Some respondents commented upon the deleterious effects of excessive talking, lecturing, threats and expressions of anger on the part of the staff. They mentioned the negative results of humiliating or teasing residents-- in other words, verbally abusing them.

When asked to comment on their total approach to the management of disruptive behavior, many respondents stressed the sig-

nificance to residents of relationships with staff--child care
staff in particular--and with peers. A planned overall approach
and skillful intervention on the part of staff were viewed as
more likely to contribute to success in coping with disruptive
behavior than the use of any particular method.

THE USE OF MEDICATION AND SECURE CONFINEMENT

In general, it has been demonstrated throughout the discussion on methods of coping with disruptive behavior that there
are potential hazards to residents in the use of any one or several of all the methods described. The special consideration
given to the use of medication and secure confinement arises out
of the unique nature of these two methods and the circumstances
under which they may be used. Both methods represent clear im-
position of external control upon an individual. Both have been
reported as used most often (with some exceptions) in instances
where a resident has either apparently lost control of his or
her actions or is in danger of doing so. A pertinent question
here might be: Is the resident "out of control of himself or is
he out of the control of the staff person?"[5]

a. Medication

Medication has been used to control or alter behavior within
the last 5 years in more than two-thirds of the responding facilities, but most describe its use as rare. Eighteen percent have
increased their use of medication in recent years because their
populations have become more disturbed, but 25% have decreased
its use because the staff has become more skilled or the population less disturbed. Medication is regarded as having the advantages of controlling behavior and making the child more accessible,
and the disadvantages of masking symptoms, becoming a crutch for
the child or the staff, or producing undesirable side effects.

The facilities in the study sample employing medication
appear, for the most part, to have instituted careful monitoring
and review procedures and to be selective in recommending this
method. They do not as a rule regard medication as a solution to
behavioral problems or symptoms but rather as a means by which a
youngster may be helped to regain control and become more accessible
to treatment. (A similar attitude exists about secure confinement
among those facilities that use it.) One would not discount the
benefits of using medication for some individuals. However, given
the increasing concern about side effects of long-term use of certain medications--psychotropic medications in particular--coupled
with what appears to be acceptance of at least some use of

medication in a large group of the facilities in this sample, the reiteration of certain cautions appears advisable.

The study findings and discussion of these data lead to the recommendation that administrators and staff of group care facilities (including their advising or attending physicians and/or psychiatrists) should include in their review of current policies and procedures regarding medication the following considerations:

. treatment goals for each resident;

. progress of individual residents, including observation of both positive and negative physical and psychosocial effects that may be attributed to use of medication;

. current information on the types of medication in use or being considered;

. alternative methods available or under consideration for residents; and

. frequency and quality of monitoring and review procedures concerning the use of medication.

b. Secure Confinement

Secure confinement has been used at some time in the last 5 years by 32 of the 144 facilities in the sample. Only four of these are group homes. Where used, confinement was estimated to have been used for a third of the residents in the last year. Authorization for confinement must usually, but not always, be obtained from the executive or a senior staff member. Secure confinement may extend beyond 24 hours in half the facilities mentioning the maximum duration. It is usually, but not always, monitored closely. Confinement is seen as helping the child regain control and preventing harm to the child or others, but, according to the respondents, it has disadvantages in that it may be abused by staff, can be psychologically harmful to the resident, and does not help the child establish long-term internal controls.

If one takes the position, as many do, that secure confinement is not desirable within the child welfare system, then a closer look at the components of "successful" alternatives may prove beneficial. If, on the other hand, one views the use of this method as necessary and/or useful as a positive intervention, the data compiled in the survey report and the example of its use given earlier point up the necessity for scrupulous consideration of all of the factors involved in employing secure confinement to manage behavior.

64

As in the case of medication, most of the small group of respondents in this survey making use of secure confinement appear to be concerned about the effects of its use, reserving the method for situations in which confining a resident is seen as a means of preventing unnecessary and/or untimely discharge. Others view its use as being of some therapeutic benefit to the resident. Differences reported in the availability of staff to a resident who is being confined show that in the majority of cases a staff member is not in constant attendance and the procedures for "monitoring" a resident do not always include the youngster's awareness that another person is around and available. In the confinement unit described earlier in this report, replacement of the one-way windows by plexiglass, through which the resident could see the staff member, was done after the one-way windows were damaged by the youngsters. Recognition of the possibilities for physical and psychological damage in completely isolating an individual, especially one who is already in a disturbed state, leads to endorsement of the policy set down in the League Standards for Services of Child Welfare Institutions:

> When isolation is selected as the most advisable form of interference, it should be handled as isolation from a situation. It is essential for the child to have an adult nearby and in contact with him.[6]

Further, any use of secure confinement should be subject to meticulous regulation and accountability both from within and outside the sponsoring facility. The employment of this measure of control must be carefully and continually reviewed by administration and staff in light of individual treatment needs. Physical safety of the resident is one paramount concern. The other, equally important, is that staff involved in implementing this method be constantly aware of the necesssity of avoiding any attitudes or actions that degrade, humiliate, or further isolate a youngster from helpful human contact in the struggle to regain control of powerful and frightening emotions.

CONCERN FOR THE CHILD CARE WORKER

In reviewing the discussion on interrelationships between behaviors and methods, residents and staff, it becomes increasingly apparent that, just as policy and programming play a significant role in outlining the course of behavior management, the actions and attitudes of line staff, particularly child care workers, are crucial.

Recognition of the need for enhancing the skills of those persons who serve as the primary agents of care for children and youths in group settings has pervaded the field for some time. Theoretical considerations and even practical justifications for doing so, often, unfortunately, become subordinate to survival issues such as lack of funding and shortage of staff.

Data gathered in this survey show a wide variation in the formal education of child care workers and the incidence of staff turnover in this position. That provision of formal in-service training other than orientation and supervision had been instituted in more than three-fourths of the responding facilities is evidence of a general effort to increase the knowledge and skill of child care workers. However, the extent of the difficulties encountered in retaining, educating and supervising child care staff on the part of the responding facilities as a whole is not known. Narrative statements from those facilities commenting on behavior management in general tended to emphasize the need for skilled intervention and the importance of the child care worker to the team. Questions concerning requests for medication and secure confinement, as well as the responsibility for implementing such methods, revealed the pivotal role of the child care worker in many instances.

Although there are theoretical and practical guidelines available regarding the incorporation of child care staff into the framework of group care and treatment,[7] individual facilities will, of course, use different resources and adopt a variety of approaches to enhance the quality and stability of care. One respondent offered a detailed set of guidelines in relation to the facility's child care staff.[8] An outline of this approach is included here as one example of the ways residential facilities define the responsibilities of both child care staff and administration.

> This facility (a residential treatment center) operates on the assumption that "acting out" on the part of residents is largely a result of deficits in the program. As an essential component of the program and prior to examining specific restrictions on a child's behavior, certain provisions should be instituted in relation to child care staff. These provisions are:
>
> Clear, written instructions defining the rules and philosophy of the facility should be given to child care workers before they begin working with residents. These instructions should include specific guidelines relating to the role of the child care worker.

. The child care worker should have the means for
immediate access to senior supervisory staff. (In
this facility access is provided through a "beeper"
page system.)

. Meetings between child care and supervisory staff
to go over what is happening in the primary group
should be scheduled regularly and frequently. Daily
meetings are recommended.

. Supervisors must provide support and nurturance to
child care workers, allowing them to express and
come to terms with their own feelings. In hiring
supervisors, facilities should seek applicants highly qualified to perform this task.

. Opportunities for formal inservice training should
be provided.

. Evaluation of child care workers should be done
annually, emphasizing individual and group goals
for the following period and the importance of the
team approach. A structured evaluation system is
recommended for all staff.

Information gathered from the 144 residential facilities in
the sample in respect to the incidence and control of disruptive behavior indicates (whether or not one subscribes to the
specifics of these guidelines or any other set of guidelines)
the importance of planful concern for child care and other line
staff cannot be stressed enough in view of the impact of the
attitudes and behavior of these adults upon the attitudes and
behavior of the children with whom they live and work.

CONCLUDING COMMENTS

Broad categorizations describing a diverse and yet select
sample of residential facilities in terms of such characteristics as size, location, staffing, programs, population served,
behavior management problems and solutions, are useful in helping to identify current trends and concerns. Not surprisingly,
however, in view of the many individual variations among the
facilities studied and the nature and scope of the survey, the
findings produced more questions than definitive answers. In
response to an apparent increase in the population of older
and more disturbed youngsters (including those labeled status
offenders, who appear, so far, to be an integral but not substantially different component of the population), the facilities in the sample reported varying degrees of success and

difficulty in behavior management. The great variety of methods employed produced no uniform set of recommended solutions to the dilemma of providing constraint without risking harm, This finding appears to support Whittaker's contention: "No single theory or set of practice prescriptions will answer the needs of a program which is geared to the total range of the child's development and oriented to the total ecology of his world."[9]

A theme frequently mentioned in this survey was the importance to residents of peer group and staff relationships, as well as the need for sound programming. The determinants of successful management of problematic behavior appeared, in the opinion of many, to be not only dependent upon the types of method used but also upon the attitudes and skills of the individuals involved in implementing them.

1. Mayer, Morris F., et al. *Group Care of Children: Crossroads and Transitions* New York: Child Welfare League of America, 1977: p.58.

2. *Ibid.* p.288.

3. *CWLA Standards for Services of Child Welfare Institutions* New Uork: Child Welfare League of America, 1964 (currently in revision).

4. Remarks concerning the study design excerpted from statement by Ralph Cordes, Field Consultant, Child Welfare League of America, at Annual Meeting of American Orthopsychiatric Association, April 1979, Washington, DC, Panel 135, "Problems of Behavior Management in Residential Settings."

5. Enders, Joseph V. and Gohe, Douglas H. "Time-Out Rooms in Residential Treatment Centers," *Child Welfare*, LII, 6 (June 1973), p.364.

6. *CWLA Standards for Services of Child Welfare Institutions* New York: Child Welfare League of America, 1964, pp.45-46.

7. See, for example, *Training for Child Care Staff* New York: Child Welfare League of America, 1963, reprinted 1978; and Lambert, Paul, *The ABCs of Child Care Work in Residential Care*, The Linden Hill Manual. New York: CWLA, 1977.

8. Excerpted from statement by Andrew Diamond, Resident Director Vista Del Mar Child Care Service, at Annual Meeting of American Orthopsychiatric Association, April 1979: Washington, DC, Panel 135, "Problems of Behavior Management in Residential Settings."

9. Whittaker, James K. "The Changing Character of Residential Child Care," *Social Service Review*, LII, p.28.

APPENDIX

Selected Excerpts from the
Survey Questionnaire

Problems

30. Please indicate the portion of your population engaging in the types of behavior listed below. In addition, for each category, check whether the incidence of that behavior at the facility has increased over the last 5 years (or since inception). If your population includes status offenders, indicate whether their presence is considered to have contributed to an increase in the incidence of each type of problematic behavior.

Type of Behavior	Proportion of Residents Involved			Check if Increased Over Last 5 Years	Check if Presence of Status Offenders Contributed to Increase
	Most	Some	None		
a. Verbal abuse directed toward children and/or adults	___	___	___	___	___
b. Physical abuse directed toward children and/or adults	___	___	___	___	___
c. Physical self-abuse	___	___	___	___	
d. Destruction of property	___	___	___	___	___
e. Disruption of the outside community	___	___	___	___	___
f. Refusal to cooperate and/or participate in the program	___	___	___	___	___
g. Refusal to go to school	___	___	___	___	___
h. Absence without leave from facility	___	___	___	___	___
i. Stealing	___	___	___	___	___
j. Use of marijuana	___	___	___	___	___
k. Use of other drugs (specify) _____	___	___	___	___	___
l. Use of alcohol	___	___	___	___	___
m. Inappropriate sexual behavior	___	___	___	___	___
n. Fire-setting	___	___	___	___	___
o. Hyperactivity	___	___	___	___	___
p. Loss of impulse control (e.g., uncontrolled outbursts)	___	___	___	___	___
q. Other behavior seen as problematic (specify) _____	___	___	___	___	___

Methods of Handling Problematic Behavior (See page 15 for instructions)

Talk - Includes discussion of any type. Discussion may be conducted with residents
         individually or in a group. The adult(s) involved may be any staff member
         including therapist, teacher, child care worker, administrator, etc., and/or
         any adult not employed by the facility.

Priv - The rescinding of privileges or rewards and/or the addition of chores or
         tasks on a short or long-term basis.

Rep   - Requiring the resident to make reparations for damage. For example, this
         would involve returning, repairing or paying for damaged, destroyed or
         stolen property, or otherwise providing just compensation.

Sep   - Separation or removal from the group--non-secure. Requires the resident to
         leave an activity or area where others are present. The resident may
         be accompanied by staff or asked to leave on his or her own. A definite
         place for removal may be specified, e.g., resident's room, a staff member's
         office, a "quiet room" or library. The resident is not locked in.

Phys - Physical restraint of the resident by one or more people in order to prevent
         harm to self, others or property.

Med   - The administering of medication to a resident for the purpose of altering
         behavior on a short or long-term basis.

Conf - Secure confinement of a resident in a locked room or unit.

Pol   - Calling the police for the purpose of subduing, arresting or locating a
         resident or group of residents.

Dis   - Discharge of a resident. Can be permanent or temporary.

Oth   - Other method(s). If the preceding categories cannot be used to describe
         your procedures in a general way, you may use this category. In Col. B or C
         define your other methods by number--e.g., "Oth 1, Oth2," etc., and explain
         them below. Feel free to add a page if you need more room.

         Oth 1: _____

         _____

         Oth 2: _____

         _____

         Oth 3: _____

         _____

Solutions

31. Column A includes a list of the types of behavior mentioned on the previous page. The opposite page describes methods of handling problematic behavior. We would like to know which methods are most often employed at your facility and what you do when your usual methods do not work and/or the situation becomes acute. Therefore, in Columns B and C, please write in the abbreviated codes for the methods you employ. You may write in as many as apply.

(For example, if for a particular behavior you most often use physical restraint and/or separation from the group, Column B would be marked "Phys," "Sep". If in extreme cases of the same behavior you would call the police and/or discharge the resident, Column C would read "Pol," "Dis".) We are aware that individual cases and methods differ greatly but would like a general response.

A Behavior	B Usual Method(s) Employed	C Method(s) Employed in Acute Situations
a. Verbal abuse of others		
b. Physical abuse of others		
c. Physical self-abuse		
d. Destruction of property		
e. Disruption of community		
f. Refusal to cooperate/ participate		
g. Refuse school		
h. Absence without leave		
i. Stealing		
j. Use of marijuana		
k. Other drugs		
l. Use of alcohol		
m. Inappropriate sexual behavior		
n. Fire-setting		
o. Hyperactivity		
p. Loss of impulse control		
q. Other (specify)_____		